Heal Your Rosacea with Essential Oils

Get Rid of Low Self Esteem with these Natural Remedies for Acne, Rosacea, Pimples (Blackheads & Whiteheads), Spider veins and Other Skin Conditions

Isabella Lily Elliott

Copyright © 2018 by Isabella Lily Elliott

All rights reserved. No part of this publication may be reproduced, distributed, or transmitted in any form or by any means, including photocopying, recording, or other electronic or mechanical methods, without the prior written permission of the publisher, except in the case of brief quotations embodied in critical reviews and certain other non-commercial uses permitted by copyright law.

Copyright © 2018 Isabella Lily Elliott

Dedication

This book is dedicated to all who desire to have a clean skin and youthful look.

Table of Content

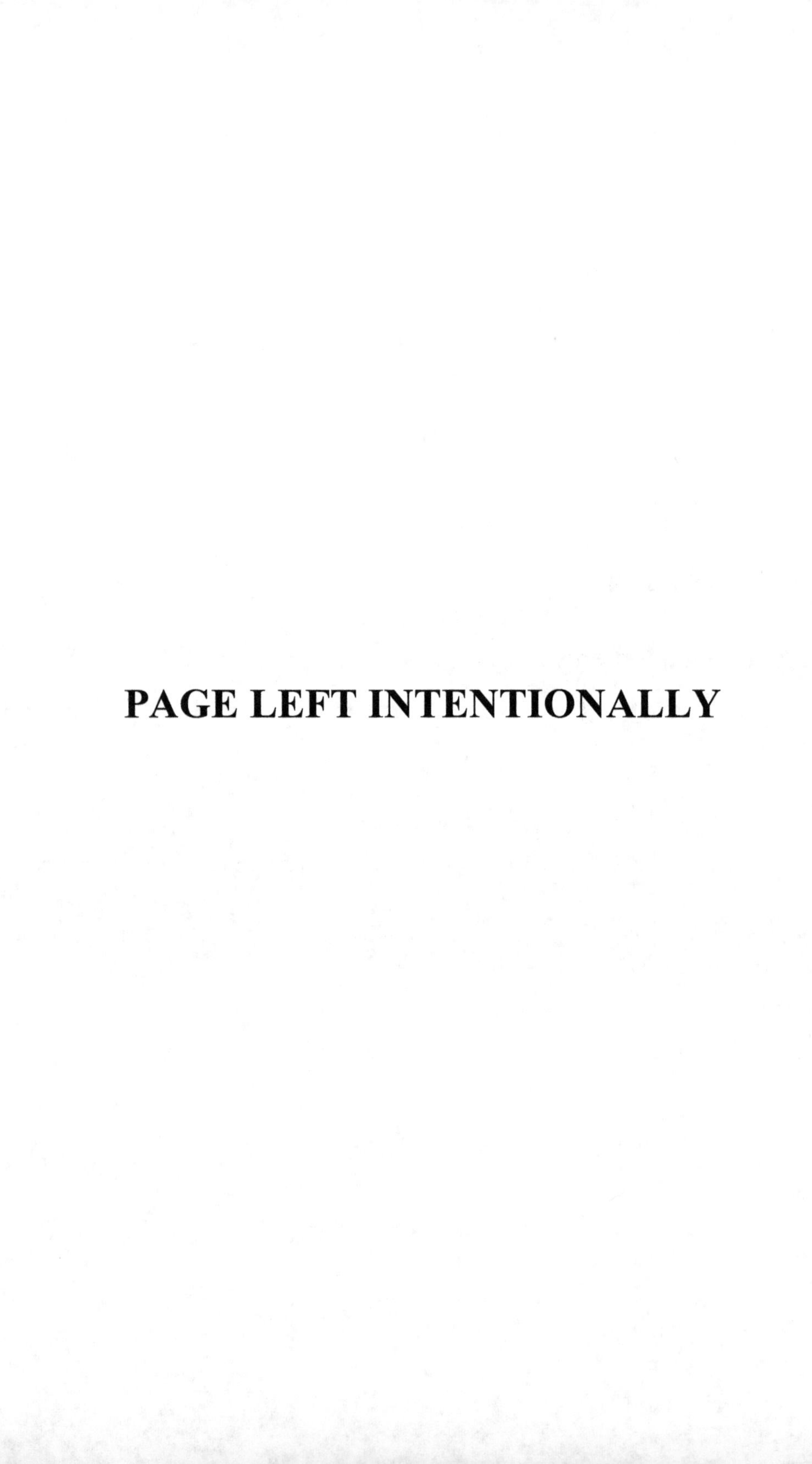

PAGE LEFT INTENTIONALLY

Introduction

Salmon Bones discovered she had this medical condition at a tender age. As years went by, the symptoms on her nose worsened and she tried severally to get a cure.

Rosacea succeeded in making her a timid and shy person as she found it difficult coming close to people for discussion. She went onto the internet to know how she could cure this skin condition and tried several medications she saw others use on the net.

Isabella took her doctor's advice to avoid triggers but the symptoms persisted.

After trying different recommendations without achieving positive result, she sought the advice of her dermatologist, she adhered strictly to the information given to her and the medication prescribed to her worked perfectly well to control the symptoms on her cheeks, chin and forehead.

She thought about laser treatment but couldn't afford it. Instead of giving up, she found alternatives to treating rosacea. She started out by using a non-alcohol toner and a cotton ball on her face twice a day. **To her surprise, not only did her pores begin to shrink, but the cysts and swelling on her nose gradually began to subside!**

This method, in combination with her dermatologists advice and prescription, her skin became a glow!

She regretted not having her treatment early enough.

To you my reader, have you been bothered so long about this skin condition of yours? Have you tried several products for this skin condition without positive result? This is the right book for you. The book contains all you need to know about rosacea, its causes, the triggers, and the natural treatments you can apply to your skin to get

the glowing skin you have always desired.

Enjoy your reading!

Chapter 1

Rosacea

What is Rosacea?

Rosacea is a skin condition that is often times misdiagnosed and misunderstood. This is because rosacea can resemble other more common skin conditions such as acne and rashes.

Rosacea happens when the blood vessels dilate, leading to redness in certain areas on the face, such as the cheekbones, the nose and the forehead.

There are lots of approach to what rosacea really is. Rosacea is generally pronounced "roh-ZAY-sha".

Generally speaking, I'll say rosacea is a chronic inflammatory disorder primarily affecting the facial skin and its mostly characterized by flare-ups and remissions.

Likewise, it is said to be a serious skin condition whereby an individual experiences persistent redness and disturbance on the central part of the face. Regularly, the cheeks are reddened. However, the condition may extend to other parts of the body like eyes, nose, brow and neck. Adults are generally affected by rosacea.

Moreover, it occurs mostly in white skinned people particularly the women.

The exact cause of this skin disease is not known. In any case, there are some signs which can indicate that an individual is affected with rosacea; which has been expressed above.

Rosacea, being a reasonably common skin issue affects about 5% of the entire population. It affects individuals who are between the ages of 20 and 40.

Mostly, it begins in the early teens and after that you have to deal with it for the rest of your life unless you make a dramatic lifestyle change or go for a professional rosacea treatment. There are numerous over the counter drugs which claim to treat rosacea, however most doctors suggest that these medicines does not work.

What causes rosacea?

Rosacea is a serious skin condition that looks like a terrible case of acne. The condition shows papules (crusty pimples), pustules (pus filled pimples), rhinophyma, bulbous, puffy cheeks and enlarged red nose.

The individual may experience greasy skin also known as seborrhea or spider veins referred to as telangiectasias. If not immediately attended to, rosacea tends to get worse.

With time the redness spreads slowly and by the age of sixty, it involves the eyes making them disturbed and ragged looking. In more extreme cases, the redness may include the nose as well because of its constant tissue use. A condition referred to as rhinophyma.

Research has revealed the disease to be caused by a few factors. Some of the investigators of the disease have linked it to the presence of bacterium helicobacter pylori which is also the cause of peptic cancer. A Japanese study has shown that sixty five percent of patients with rosacea had this microorganism. Be that as it may, the study involved seventy percent of the whole population.

It would appear as if the bacterium is not the cause of the disease, but an antibody that is associated with the killing of helicobacter pylori was found in one hundred percent of the patients that recovered completely, from the treatment of rosacea by use of antibiotics.

These results are confusing because they suggest that the bacterium is not the cause of the disease, but killing the bacterium cures the individual from rosacea disease. Most of the physicians treating rosacea sufferers avoid endorsing antibiotics and only resort to it on short term basis in extreme cases.

Another investigation linked the cause of rosacea to Demodex follicularum, which is a type of house mite. The house mite is a microscopic spider relative that usually resides in healthy skin and feeds on sebum, the oil secreted by the skin. It is commonly noticed first under the eyelashes. A person with these mites under their eyes suffers from burning eyes, sticky eyes and itches.

The microscopic mite also lives on the face, cheeks, forehead, on the external ear channel and anywhere on dogs. It is the cause of mange in dogs.

Some medical books explain that the disease is common in cold climates where people often get red faces due to the cold weather. However, exposure to the sunlight is just as possible to cause rosacea as exposure to the cold. In actual fact, the dry weather poses more severe problems. According to these researchers, people with rosacea have sun damaged skin. Normally the connective tissues are broken and loose, they are not capable of supporting the blood vessels hence allow inflammatory cytokines to accumulate and cause flare-ups.

In addition to these factors is stress. When people are stressed, the nerve cells on the skin break open releasing adrenaline and substance P.

Substance P reaches the skin through the bloodstream and increases the growth and productivity of the cells that produces oil. This way, a considerable measure of oil is poured out into the follicles helping with rosacea treatment.

Things that triggers Rosacea

You may have likely noticed that certain foods, temperatures, activities, emotions -- or something else entirely -- will trigger your rosacea to breakout. Listed below are some common rosacea triggers.

1. Foods and drinks that cause rosacea

i.   Alcohol

ii.   Spicy foods

iii.   Hot drinks

iv.   Hot foods (in temperature)

v.   Activities that cause rosacea:

vi.   Exercise or heavy exertion

vii.   Hot baths or saunas

2. Weather conditions that cause rosacea

i.   Hot weather

ii.   Cold weather

iii.   Humid weather

iv.   Wind

v.   Sunlight

3. Emotions that cause rosacea

i.   Stress or anxiety

ii.   Sudden change in emotion, like feeling embarrassed or bursting out laughing

4. Medical conditions that cause rosacea

i.   Menopause

ii.   Chronic cough

iii.   Caffeine withdrawal syndrome

5. Other rosacea triggers

i.   Skin products

ii.   Medications, such as topical steroids, some blood pressure drugs, and some opiate painkillers.

Please note that, it is not all the mentioned triggers that can cause rosacea. Everyone has got different immune system. The important thing is to learn what causes your own rosacea symptoms. You can use a diary to keep track.

Whenever you notice a change in your skin, keep tab of what you ate or drank. Be aware of things you do so as to know what primarily triggered the skin condition.

Chapter 2

Sub-types of Rosacea

According to the symptoms, rosacea is divided into four subtypes:

Subtype 1 (erythematotelangiectatic rosacea), portrayed by flushing and persistent redness, and may also incorporate visible blood vessels.

Subtype 2 (papulopustular rosacea), portrayed by persistent redness with transient bumps and pimples.

Subtype 3 (phymatous rosacea), portrayed by skin thickening, often resulting in an enlargement of the nose from excess tissue.

Subtype 4 (ocular rosacea), portrayed by ocular manifestations, for example; dry eye, tearing and burning, swollen eyelids, recurrent styes and potential vision loss from corneal damage.

How to prevent Rosacea

Though there are no actual cure for rosacea, but there are many effective treatment in the market which range from surgical procedures to creams and ointments.

The actual cause of rosacea is unknown, but there are ways to help prevent it. Some of the prevention methods include:

1. Using a mild cleanser: Use a liquid facial purifier that has disodium lauryl sulfosuccinate or sodium lauryl sulfate. These ingredients will clean your

pores and skin lightly without giving you irritations that would cause flushing.

2. Soothe your skin with chamomile: Almost everyone knows chamomile to be a soothing relief for rosacea-susceptible skin. It is therefore advisable to use moisturizers, soaps and cleansers which contains chamomile, an herb in the ragweed family. However, if you know you are allergic to ragweed, please stay away from cleansers that contains chamomile.

3. Avoiding harsh sunlight: Stay out of hot sunlight. The sun could be so up that no amount of sunscreen will cover up for the burns.

4. Keeping away from abrasives: It's ideal you avoid abrasives as much as you can. Getting in contact with this can cause a flush. Stay away from cleansers and scrubs that contains such.

5. Cucumber moisturizer: Using moisturizers that contains cucumber extracts is good for the skin. Cleaning the skin lightly with this moisturizer cleans your pores and skin. It has been reported that cucumber creams soothe rosacea-prone skin.

6. Sunscreen: It is important you use the best of titanium dioxide sunscreen everytime you are outdoor. Avoid every other chemical sunscreens and keep only those that contains titanium dioxide as its most important ingredients. This sunscreen soothes rosacea-prone skin.

7. Wearing cool clothes: It is important you wear mild clothes to keep the body cool always. Take cool baths and showers as well. Avoid wool clothings too. Wool tends to cause redness and rashness especially to those who are at risk of rosacea.

8. Be mindful of what you eat: Watching your diet intake and identifying food allergies. Avoid spicy foods that triggers rosacea. Stay away from foods that contains tobasco sauce, chilli peppers, and horseradish. It is also necessary you stay away from chocloate, and carbonated drinks.

9. Take more of vegetables: Consume more of dark greens like kale, spinach, broccoli and asparagus. These veggies contain high vitamin A and C, bioflavonoids and beta-carotene. They help to strenghten the body capillaries and boost the immune system.

10. Avoid alcohol: The consumption of alcohols triggers the blood vessels within the body system and causes the skin pores to dilate making rosacea to appear in an individual.

With all these said, to identify the triggers, you may want to write down each time an attack happens and what you were doing and eating or drinking at the time. Rosacea treatments work for some people while others do not respond at all. You may need to experiment with the different products available to find the one that works right for you.

Chapter 3

Symptoms of rosacea

This self-conscious inflicting condition normally affects individuals in different forms. In some persons, it could be;

1. Redness of the central face, over the nose, forehead, and cheeks

2. Redness affecting the chest, neck, scalp and ears

3. The facial blood vessels may dilate and amplify close to the skin surface.

4. Experiencing semi-permanent redness, red grainy eyes, red domed papules and pustules

5. Throbbing and burning sensations, and in most outrageous cases,

6. A red swollen nose.

Other symptoms of rosacea

Other symptoms of rosacea include;

1. Red zones either across or on certain spots on your face.

2. Tiny, red bumps, mostly known as pustules on your cheeks, nose, jaw and forehead may also form. This should not be confused with blackheads or clogged pores.

3. Noticeable and perceivable blood vessels on your cheeks and nose.

4. Propensity to redden or flush quite effortlessly.

5. Burning or grainy feeling in your eyes, which poses a great concern if it ever occurs.

6. Rhinophyma or having a large, red, inflamed nose.

7. Broken blood vessels which are visible.

8. Dryness of skin,

There are some auxiliary features that can be classified into extra rosacea symptoms. Your facial skin may progress towards becoming extremely dry, it may exhibit lifted red patches, it may start to sting, your face may appear puffy, and the skin could severely thicken.

These symptoms could likewise appear on any other part of the body.

Rosacea can quite be a harmless condition for some, however in the event that it gets aggrevated, it can not only turn out to become a severe cosmetic condition for your face, yet also an enormous self-esteem demolisher. The side effects of rosacea such as the ones mentioned above can be avoided by some of the most common prevention techniques out there.

Chapter 4

How severe is your Rosacea?

Having rosacea can be easily determined provided you have the basic information about it. Rosacea appears in stages and you can easily tell which stage you fall into.

Stage 1: Vulgaris

This is the stage of rosacea that everyone would be aware of. This stage is commonly seen in teens at the onset of puberty, due to hormonal changes in the body. The common appearance of the skin blemish come in the following forms:

- Blackheads

- Whiteheads

- Papules - obvious red areas which appear higher than the surrounding skin

- Pustules - Lumps containing pus

Stage 2: Acne Rosacea

This is a type of rosacea condition which appears as a red rash and is seen on the skin between pimples and other types of blemishes commonly associated with vulgaris sufferers. However, this condition is not normally seen in women as much as it is seen in the male population.

Stage 3: Conglobata

This stage can lead to permanent scarring so the recommendation is to visit your health professional. This normally appears as linked sores that are full of whiteheads, blackheads and sores.

Stage 4: Fulminans

This can be likened to conglobata, however this type of rosacea will develop very quickly. This type is commonly seen in men, one of the side effects is aching of the muscles and body joints.

Again, medical attention would be re□uired if you are suffering from this type of acne.

Medical practitioners would normally treat this form of acne with a drug call Accutane. However, like all drugs, there are side effects which I would suggest you do a little research on if these drugs were prescribed to you. Pregnant women ought to be cautious with respect to this drug.

Stage 5: Pyroderma Faciale

This is another form of rosacea which can lead to permanent scarring if not treated early. The good news for men...it is normally seen in women in the age group of 20's, 30's and 40's. Sufferers will have a very painful

experience with nodules and sores.

Chapter 5

How to treat Rosacea

There are numerous treatment easily accessible for rosacea, however there is no established cure for rosacea. The mainstay treatment for rosacea consists of oral and topical antibiotics.

However, proceeding with the use of antibiotics can cause antibiotic resistance. The most validated topical therapies include metronidazole, azelaic acid, and sodium sulfacetamide-sulfur. Other topical therapies, such as calcineurin inhibitors, benzoyl peroxide, clindamycin, retinoids, topical corticosteroids, and permethrin have revealed unpredictable degrees of achievements.

Many rosacea sufferers discover standard treatments are insufficient or even exacerbating. Due to the inconsistent results of drug treatments, rosacea sufferers are increasingly interested in alternative therapies using natural products to ease inflammation and alleviate rosacea.

The Natural Treatment for Rosacea

The rosacea natural treatment is probably the only method in existence, to permanently eliminate the condition, and all its symptoms. It is based on the fact that roughly 94% of rosacea patients lack a certain amino-acid, which is available in healthy people.

Taking supplements with the amino-acid, or simply eating foods rich in it immediately makes the symptoms and redness vanish.

In addition, in the event that you go to a physician/doctor, you will usually get a prescription for a moisturizing skin lotion, and be told that the condition is completely harmless, and affects a lot of people. I'm positive that is not what you want to hear.

Some doctors are actually a bit more concerned, and prescribe special lotions, designed for the condition. This rarely works either, because the problem is still present - you lack the protein, necessary in collagen, and pigmentation synthesis. That is why the rosacea natural treatment is so effective - it simply treats the root cause, making the symptoms quickly disappear, usually in a matter of a few days.

Generally speaking, rosacea is harmless. Be that as it may, it can cause most people a lot of suffering, low self-esteem, and less socializing. That's especially true in women, which are most commonly influenced with the condition, sometimes because of genetics, and sometimes because of their poor diets, aimed at keeping certain body-weight. Whatever may be the cause, the condition can be treated naturally, and cured □uickly.

What you need to know is that rosacea is caused by your own body. Once you give your body what it wants, it instantly settles the condition on its own. The store-bought lotions do not do that, and are usually made for a very temporary relief of the redness, as well as a covering effect, much like make up.

Those solutions are really short-term and are useless. The only way to treat the condition, is to remove the underlying cause, which can be accomplished very

☐uickly, provided that you know what you are doing.

There are several natural ways to cure your rosacea

naturally. The most easiest and effective rosacea cure is

1. By simply taking care of your skin. Sufferers are advised to clean their face with a gentle and non-abrasive cleanser, then wash with lukewarm water and pat the face dry using a soft cotton towel. Do not tug, pull or use a rough washcloth.

2. The next thing to do is to wear a sunscreen with an SPF factor of 15 or greater to protect the skin from sun exposure.

3. Consuming natural products would certainly be a better option than prescription medications. One of the natural ways to cure rosacea is to make green tea paste at your home. Grind some green tea leaves and add water or milk to make a paste out

of it approximately which can be used for two days. Apply it on the affected parts of your face and leave for 10-15 minutes. The green tea has a soothing property that helps the redness. Over a couple of days, you should notice a significant improvement in your condition.

4. You can also apply vinegar on the rosacea sites but you have to allow it settle. You have to allow it get deep which implies you should keep for at least one hour. Apple cider vinegar has been sworn by many to be highly effective in rosacea cure and numerous other skin conditions.

5. You can also apply moderate amount of aloe vera gel on the affected area. It helps to minimize redness, itching, and also it can effectively cure the rosacea.

6. Other effective natural cures for rosacea include oatmeal which helps to provide a barrier to reduce moisture loss when applied twice a day to the affected regions.

These are the most important things to do while trying to cure rosacea. Above all, believe in yourself and stay positive.

Chapter 6

Fundamental conditions that can cause Rosacea

As a lot of research is still in progress in order to find out what might be the actual cause of rosacea. However, here are some points that might contribute to this condition.

1. **Genes:** Rosacea is understood to be a family phenomenon, which means, there is possibility for it to be passed down to any of the children if possessed by either of the parents. So, it can be genetic most times.

2. **H pylori bug:** This bug is known to have the ability of causing infection to the intestine, and it can also have a role in causing rosacea to the body.

Researchers have found that many people with rosacea have pylori infections, but it cannot be proved that it causes it directly, as many people without rosacea also have H pylori infections.

3. **Bacteria***:* Science has found that most people with the acne-like version of rosacea have an overactive immune response to a bacterium called oleronius. Though, scientists are not sure if this may be a clue to the immune system role in the condition.

4. **Mites***:* The living organism known as Demodex, is a mite that is present on every human's skin might also be a cause of rosacea. These mites live on the cheeks and nose, which is largely where rosacea shows up. Studies have shown that, there are numerous numbers of these mites living in the skin of everyone that has rosacea. However, these mites are also present on non-rosacea patient'sskin too,

which makes it hard to say this is a definite cause of the condition.

5. **Protein***:* Cathelicidin is a protein that normally protects our skin from common infections, but it could be the cause of swelling and redness in people with rosacea. The way the body processes the protein could be causing the condition.

Chapter 7

Supplements that causes Rosacea

In most cases, these supplements may activate facial redness, facial flushing and rosacea outbreaks without the rosacea sufferer even having the idea of the source of the rosacea trigger due to the fact that there may be some differences in time between taking the oral supplement and the supplement triggering vascular hyper-reactivity in the facial region — this lag time may take as long as 8 to 12 hours — thus making it very difficult to identify oral supplements as triggers.

However, there are several supplements taken by many people and are ignorant of the fact that these supplements may directly of indirectly cause rosacea. Some of these supplements include:

1. ***Coenzyme Q10:*** This is a potent dilator that mostly cause rosacea flushing. The wisest approach to taking this supplement is to take 50 mg daily for two to four weeks to let your body acclimate to the supplement (the average starting dose is 100 to 200 mg). Don't rush it and be sure to take note of the number of times you flush or flare to determine if it is safe for you to continue taking this supplement.

2. ***Green Tea Extract:*** This is usually an effective supplement for rosacea sufferers due to its anti-inflammatory actions and skin-specific incorporation into the dermis. The main disadvantage of taking this supplement is that many rosacea sufferers take 500 mgs to 750 mgs

which is well above the recommended dose and can cause tachycardia (high heart rate) and high blood pressure — both worsen rosacea symptoms.

3. ***Ginko Biloba:*** Ginkgo biloba has been used medicinally for thousands of years. It is a potent dilator and increases cognitive abilities in the brain due to the delivery of nutrients and oxygen. This is an excellent supplement, however it fre□uently causes flushing, even at the lowest concentrations. It is best to find alternative ways to enhance cognition as this is usually too much for rosacea sufferers.

Other supplements include; "L-Arginine and L-Citrulline" & "High doses of Amino Acids and Protein".

Dietary Triggers & Help

Whilst there are numerous dietary triggers for sufferers of rosacea and they will vary from person to person, alcohol and spicy foods are among the two most commonly reported, and individuals who have cut these out of their diet often find that flare ups are significantly reduced. Other common food triggers include the following;

1. Chocolate

2. Soy sauce

3. Yeast extract

4. Some beans and pods, including lima, navy or peas

5. Caffeine

6. Sugar and processed foods

7. Conventional dairy products

8. Fried foods, hydrogenated oils, Trans fats.

People who do not decide to make modifications to their meal and lifestyle always find that they struggle to keep-up a good nutritional balance.

Those who do not feel confident about actualizing changes independently may benefit from the expertise of a qualified nutritionist, who will ensure that whilst some food is removed they will be substituted with another. As well as giving you a personalized nutrition routine, a nutritionist will also guide you through the process, giving you motivation and support.

Supplements beneficial for healthy skin, hair, eyelashes & nails.

Are you disturbed with dry skin, cracked lips, or dull hair? Natural dietary supplements or vitamins for hair and skin may be the answer you're looking for. But while there are no shortage of vitamins for skin and hair in the market, not everyone of them are created equal.

1. **Let's look at biotin**: One of the hair vitamins found in many foods and available over the counter in supplement form at pharmacies and grocery stores, also good for keeping a healthy skin. Some reasearches show that cigarette smoking may cause a deficiency in biotin, with symptoms that includes:

I. Loss of hair color;

II. Red scaly rash around the eyes, nose, and mouth;

III. Thinning of the hair;

Biotin could be the hair growth vitamin you've been looking for. As with any vitamin for skin or hair, always consult with your physician before you try it.

2. **Omega-3 fatty acid:** This is another vitamin for hair and skin. This vitamin may boost the shine in your hair and keep your tender scalp from flaking. Recommended for a healthy skin and hair growth.

3. **Zinc:** Zinc also has antioxidant properties and is vital to your body's resistance to infection and for tissue repair. High doses of zinc are harmful though, so talk to your doctor about your diet to see if you need to supplement.

4. **Vitamin C:** This is another vitamin for skin as it helps your skin retain collagen, providing it with a smoother appearance. Many hair vitamins and vitamins for skin have the power to give you a younger-looking complexion, shinier strands, and

stronger nails. Just make sure to check with a doctor before adding any of these supplements to your routine.

5. **Iron:** Iron isn't a vitamin – it's a mineral that carries oxygen through the body, and it's necessary for the growth of healthy hair and nails.

Proper ways of maintaining the skin

At the point when people think of beauty care, they instantly think of skin, hair, and nails. In the event that you ask a group of people, which is more important to one's personal beauty care routine, you will get a variety of answers, with responses being more than likely e☐ual amounts of people valuing skin, hair, and nails.

Their response would neither be wrong nor right. However, everyone should regularly maintain their body and in doing so aids in the maintenance of the skin, hair, and nails.

A healthy up-keep program for one's body is eating a nutritional diet, refraining from smoking and drug use, reducing alcohol intake, regular exercise, ample rest, drink plenty of water, and getting plenty of (protected) sun and fresh air. This will improve the condition and health of your skin, hair, and nails from the inside out. This lays a great foundation for proper skin, hair, and nail care routines.

Your skin should receive a little extra attention due to the fact that it is the largest organ in your body, and it is your shield of armor. If you do not do your part in protecting your shield of armor, which is your skin, it cannot effectively protect you and will begin to show the signs of damage from fighting the elements alone.

Your skin care routine does not have to be expensive nor extensive, just done on a regular schedule. Be cautious when choosing your skin care products. Many skin care products in the market today are made with toxic chemicals that can cause serious harm over use.

Skin care products do not re□uire approval from the U.S. Food and Drug Administration (FDA) nor is there any check standard for quality or proof of claim of benefits. Often times the claims of benefits of skin care products are greatly exaggerated.

One way to choose □uality products is by word of mouth from friends and families to see what has worked well for them. However, the fact that one product may have worked for their skin type and conditions does not necessarily mean it will work the same way for you. Another more effective option is to consult with an aesthetician. An aesthetician can help you pick out skin care products specific for your particular skin needs. They have access to skin care products that you would be made available to you, and they usually know the outcome of the latest medical studies.

Skin care products should include quality sun protection. Some skin care products come already with a sun protection factor. An aesthetician can help you to determine which sun protection method will be most productive for you. You should be sure the cream protects you from both UVA and UVB rays since both may be harmful to the skin.

Nail care and hair care are just as essential as far as appearance value is to your skin. However, skin care does hold a bit more precedence over the two. An aesthetician can also help you in the selection of other products that lack harmful chemicals. A nail tech can guide you through a healthy nail care routine to minimize the risks of fungal and antibiotic resistant staph infections.

They can also share tips with you on proper cuticle and nail care. Indeed, you should always maintain your skin just like you would do to your hair and nails if not even more so, after all, it is the only one you have and keeping it healthy should be second nature to us all.

Chapter 8

Essential oils for Rosacea

Essential oils are effective oils used for treating skin inflammations, also used for preventing future outbreaks of rosacea. Below are some effective ones which could come handy when needed.

I.   Lavender Oil

II.   Geranium Oil

III.   Borage Oil

IV.   German Chamomile Oil

V.   Tea Tree Oil

VI.   Helichrysum Oil

VII.   Neroli Oil

VIII.   Oregano Oil

IX.   Sea Buckthorn Oil

X.   Bergamot Oil

XI.   Rosehip Oil

XII. Jojoba Oil

The Efficacy of Tea Tree Oil and Apple cider Vinegar for Rosacea

This should be aplied on a cotton ball as toner on the affected part early in the morning and night.

Ingredients:

1 cup ACV

2 cups water

5 drops tea tree oil

Method:

1. Add all ingredients in a jar and seal tightly.

2. Apply daily and night by putting it on a cotton ball and swipe your face liberally. The mixture will dry up and clear up few pimples immediately, leaving few areas dry.

3. Next step is to add a dab of cotton ball with a tiny bit of ACV and soak it with water and moisturize with the diluted EVOO. This will leave your face so soft and acne free.

4. Repeat this process day and night for three days, if you notice changes in your skin continue using it for the next seven days. But if no change is noticed on the third day, I strongly advise you to stop the process, as you know our body differs.

Avoiding outbreaks and re-lapses

The best results for this problematic skin condition during re-lapses and outbreaks is through the use of rosacea skincare products that protects and moisturizes as they reduce redness and soothe and calm the inflammatory response associated with rosacea.

These outbreaks also make changes with your lifestyle; in the sense that you become watchful of what you use and the kind of diet you consume.

The first step of preventing this re-occurence is by having a thorough skin evaluation to analyze and diagnose the condition. Once the diagnosis of rosacea is established during a professional skin consultation, medical grade rosacea skincare products may be prescribed by a ☐ualified practitioner.

Centers specializing in the treatment of problem skin disorders, skin rejuvenation and anti-aging skincare provides the best treatment options for those with rosacea.

Conclusion

Rosacea is actually a very common condition that affects millions of people every single day. In some cases, the symptoms are so minor that you are not required to do much, other than using a topical cream from time to time. Sometimes, and for many people, the symptoms are serious enough that further rosacea treatment will be needed.

Whether you are having a rosacea outbreak or not, it is important that you always use proper skincare and natural approaches as explained above to help manage rosacea and mitigate the development and recurrence of flare-ups. You can never ignore your facial skin, and removing harsh or abrasive ingredients into your skin care regimen is of paramount importance.

Prioritize skincare products that are safe, mild, and effective at taking care of your face without causing issues.

If you do have rosacea flare-ups, consult your doctor in order to determine the best approach to get your skin back to normal as soon as possible.

About The Author

Isabella Lily Elliott is a Dermatologist with over ten years of experience diagnosing and treating variety of skin conditions.

She is proficient in a variety of treatments, including laser therapy and injecting Botox safely.

She has successfully counselled many who suffered from several skin conditions.

She is a mother, wife and a community leader.

Acknowledgement

This book is dedicated to my niece, Salman bones. I love to see your smooth skin over and over again.

www.ingramcontent.com/pod-product-compliance
Lightning Source LLC
Chambersburg PA
CBHW060210260726

48658CB00005BA/1971